Real Food's Fertility Power

A Handbook on Preparing Your Body for Pregnancy through Preconception Nutrition and Fertility Awareness Methods

Jessica W. Brown

1

TABLE OF CONTENTS

INTRODUCTION

Welcome to the journey of Real Food's fertility power, where nourishment meets natural wisdom on the path to parenthood. In today's fast-paced world and ever-changing healthcare landscape, the hunt for fertility can often feel daunting and overwhelming. Yet, within the simple yet profound act of fueling our bodies with real, wholesome foods, a transformational potential awaits to be unleashed.

In this book, we go on an adventure of investigation and discovery, led by the conviction that the food we eat has the power to alter our reproductive journey in ways we never imagined. Drawing on cutting-edge scientific research, time-honored traditions, and personal experiences, we'll dig into the fascinating world of fertility nutrition and learn how to harness the healing power of real food to improve reproductive health and enhance the likelihood of conception.

However, Real Food's fertility power is more than just nutritional advice; it is a celebration of the extraordinary relationship between nourishment and conception, a monument to our bodies' natural wisdom, and a light of hope for those embarking on the path to parenthood. Whether you're just starting on your fertility journey, navigating the ups and downs of assisted reproductive technologies, or looking for natural ways to boost fertility, this book will help and empower you every step of the way. So join us on this nourishing journey, where each meal is an opportunity to heal our bodies, acknowledge our fertility, and embrace the amazing potential of genuine food to fuel our dreams of parenting. Let us work together to unleash food's transforming potential and lay the groundwork for the lovely trip that awaits us.

CHAPTER 1

WHAT IS ACTUAL FOOD FOR FERTILITY?

Real food for fertility is a dietary approach that emphasizes complete, nutrient-dense foods to promote reproductive health and fertility. Unlike processed and refined foods, which are frequently depleted of natural nutrients and loaded with additives, real foods are unprocessed and include a wealth of vitamins, minerals, antioxidants, and other critical nutrients required for reproductive health.

Here's a detailed look at what defines the actual diet for fertility:
Colorful fruits and vegetables provide the backbone of a fertility-friendly diet. They are high in vitamins, minerals, and antioxidants, which help reduce inflammation, maintain hormonal balance, and protect reproductive cells from oxidative damage. Leafy greens like spinach, kale, and Swiss chard are especially advantageous because of their high folate content, which is required for good egg and sperm production.

Whole grains, including quinoa, brown rice, oats, and barley, contain complex carbs, fiber, and vital elements such as B vitamins and magnesium. These nutrients help to manage blood sugar levels, boost energy generation, and maintain overall reproductive health.

Choosing whole grains over processed grains helps to regulate hormone levels and maintain a healthy weight, both of which are crucial in fertility.

Lean Proteins: Lean protein sources include poultry, fish, eggs, lentils, and tofu, which are necessary for tissue development and repair, including reproductive tissues. Protein is also important for fertility since it helps with hormone production and regulation. Lean proteins help lower saturated fat intake while also providing high-quality nutrients free of needless chemicals and hormones.

Healthy Fats: Healthy fats are necessary for hormone production and reproductive health. Avocados, almonds, seeds, olive oil, and fatty fish such as salmon and mackerel are also good sources of healthful fat. Omega-3 fatty acids are particularly crucial for sperm health, egg quality, and inflammation reduction in the body. Incorporating these fats into your diet can aid with fertility and enhance the likelihood of conception.

Dairy and dairy alternatives, such as almond milk, coconut yogurt, and cashew cheese, can be included in a fertility-friendly diet, particularly if they are low in added sugars and saturated fats. Dairy products contain calcium, vitamin D, and other nutrients that are beneficial to bone health and reproductive function. Some people may prefer dairy alternatives due to lactose sensitivity or dietary choices.

Herbs and Spices: Certain herbs and spices have long been used to promote reproductive health and conception. Ginger, turmeric, cinnamon, and garlic are examples of anti-inflammatory foods that may aid in menstrual cycle regulation and sperm quality improvement. Incorporating these herbs and spices into your cooking can enhance the flavor and nutritional value of your food.

Hydration: Proper hydration is critical for good health and fertility. Water serves to maintain body temperature, carry nutrients to cells, and remove toxins from the body. It also promotes cervical mucus synthesis, which is necessary for sperm survival and movement. Drinking plenty of water and herbal teas throughout the day can help you stay hydrated and promote reproductive health.

Real food for fertility promotes entire, nutrient-dense foods that contain the key nutrients required to maintain reproductive health and fertility. Individuals can naturally nourish their bodies and boost their chances of conception by eating fruits, vegetables, whole grains, lean proteins, healthy fats, and herbs/spices. Staying hydrated and limiting your intake of processed and refined foods might also help with fertility.

CHAPTER 2

THE FERTILITY CHALLENGE

Fertility problems are complicated and multidimensional concerns that can impact people or couples who are attempting to conceive. These issues can be caused by a range of reasons, including biological, environmental, lifestyle, and medical disorders. Understanding the nature of reproductive difficulties is critical for people pursuing parenting.

Biological Factors: Fertility falls as people age due to changes in reproductive hormones and the quality of their eggs and sperm. Women are born with a limited number of eggs, and as women age, the amount and quality of their eggs diminish, resulting in lower fertility and an increased risk of miscarriage. Similarly, sperm quality and quantity may deteriorate with aging, reducing male fertility. Hormonal abnormalities, such as irregular menstrual cycles, polycystic ovarian syndrome (PCOS), and thyroid diseases, can all interfere with ovulation and conception in women. Men's sperm production and motility may be affected by hormonal abnormalities, such as testosterone levels.

Reproductive Disorders: Endometriosis, uterine fibroids, blocked fallopian tubes, and male factor infertility concerns such as varicocele or erectile dysfunction can all limit reproduction.

Environmental and lifestyle factors: Environmental Toxins: Exposure to pollutants, toxins, and chemicals in the air, water, and food supply can impair fertility by changing hormone levels, causing reproductive organ damage, and decreasing sperm and egg quality. Chronic stress can interfere with reproductive hormones and interrupt menstrual cycles in women, while it can impair sperm production and motility in males.

High amounts of stress can also have an impact on libido and sexual function, hindering fertility. Diet and Nutrition: Poor dietary habits, such as eating processed foods, drinking too much alcohol, smoking, and being overweight, can hurt fertility by causing hormonal imbalances, inflammation, and oxidative stress. In contrast, a diet high in whole foods, antioxidants, and critical nutrients can help with reproductive health and fertility.

Medical conditions and treatments: Diabetes, autoimmune illnesses, obesity, and cancer are examples of medical conditions that can interfere with hormone levels, ovulation, or sperm production and hence impact fertility. Chronic health issues may need medications or therapies that influence fertility.

Assisted Reproductive Technologies (ART): When natural conception is not possible or successful, individuals may use ART methods such as in vitro fertilization (IVF), intrauterine insemination (IUI), or egg/sperm donation to produce pregnancy. While these treatments might give couples struggling with infertility hope, they can also be costly, emotionally draining, and physically demanding.

Navigating fertility issues may be a very personal and emotional process, fraught with uncertainty, frustration, and sadness. However, it is also a journey of resilience, hope, and tenacity, as people and couples consider numerous alternatives, seek assistance, and make lifestyle adjustments to improve their chances of conception. Individuals can empower themselves to walk the transforming journey to parenting by knowing the nuances of fertility issues and addressing them with compassion, information, and holistic techniques.

CHAPTER 3

BEST FOODS TO EAT WHEN YOU'RE TRYING TO CONCEIVE

Now that you're trying to conceive now is a great time to focus on healthy eating habits. Here are the meals and nutrients you need the most right now. You don't have to wait until you're pregnant to begin eating healthy. In reality, eating a nutritious diet before you conceive can help increase your fertility, lower your risk of birth defects like spina bifida, and even lessen your odds of having preeclampsia during pregnancy.

Important nutrients to consume when attempting to conceive.

As a pregnant woman, you'll need a variety of nutritious foods, such as Folic acid and folate This B vitamin (B9) is one of the most critical elements to consume before (and during) pregnancy. According to the Centers for Disease Control and Prevention (CDC), all women of reproductive age should ingest 400 micrograms (mcg) per day to help prevent neural tube disorders like spina bifida and anencephaly. To be safe, your prenatal vitamin should contain 400 to 600 mcg of folate or folic acid (the synthetic type). Foods containing folate and folic acid include Green vegetables with leaves. Spinach, broccoli, bok choy, Swiss chard, and kale are also suitable possibilities. Sauté in olive oil and serve as a side dish, or add to soups, salads, casseroles, and omelets.

Cereals with added vitamins and minerals. Look for breakfast cereals that have 100% of the daily recommended value. Strawberry with oranges. These are delicious and simple to integrate into your diet! Soybeans and nuts. Consuming beans and nuts, which are high in fiber, can also help keep you regular.

Calcium: Calcium keeps your reproductive system running normally and may even help you get pregnant sooner. It's critical to stock up now because your baby's teeth and bone health and growth will depend on a consistent supply. If your calcium levels are low when pregnant, your body will remove it from your bones and give it to the developing baby, increasing your risk of osteoporosis (brittle bones) in the future.

Get about 1,500 milligrams (mg) of calcium per day from sources like Milk. One cup of milk, the most popular calcium source, contains 299 mg, or around one-third of the daily required amount. It also has a sprinkle of vitamin D. Soy milk, almond milk, and calcium-fortified juice all contain calcium.

Drink a glass as a snack or as the foundation for a smoothie. Yogurt. One cup of plain yogurt contains about 415 mg, which is roughly one-third of your daily recommended consumption. It, like milk, can be eaten straight or topped with fruit, or it can serve as the foundation for a smoothie.

Cheese. A 1.5-ounce portion of mozzarella contains 333 mg of calcium, an equal-sized meal of cheddar contains 307 mg, and one cup of cottage cheese contains 138 mg. Kale and broccoli are two vegetables. These vegetables are high in calcium and are not dairy products.

Iron: This mineral, which transports oxygen throughout your body, will also play a crucial role in oxygen delivery to your kid. If you're having a preconception checkup, ask your doctor if you should be evaluated for iron deficiency, as too little iron may raise your baby's chance of being underweight or early. Women require approximately 18 mg per day, but your daily iron requirement increases to 27 mg per day while pregnant. Keep in mind that your body absorbs iron better through diet.

Good sources include: Breakfast cereals are fortified. One dish of fortified breakfast cereal has 18 mg of iron. Lean meat. Beef, chicken, and turkey all have approximately 1 mg of iron per 3 oz serving. Spinach. ½ cup of cooked, drained spinach has 3 mg of iron per serving, which is approximately 17% of the daily required consumption. Omega-3 Fatty Acids Although many prenatal supplements contain omega-3 fatty acids, it's also crucial to eat plenty of healthy foods while attempting to conceive.

Omega-3 fatty acids may assist regulate critical ovulation-inducing hormones while also increasing blood supply to the reproductive organs. You can locate them in Seafood. Fish heavy in fat, such as salmon, anchovies, sardines, and herring, are excellent providers of omega-3s. Grass-fed beef. Beef from grass-fed cows provides more omega-3s than grain-fed cows. Nuts and seeds. Omega-3 fatty acids can be found in walnuts, flaxseed, and chia seeds, as well as plant oils such as flaxseed, soybean, and canola. For added crunch, mix them into your smoothie or sprinkle them on top of a salad. Fiber Including more complex, slowly digesting carbs like fiber in your diet will keep you feeling fuller for longer.

Furthermore, one study found that increasing your fiber intake by 10 grams per day can reduce your risk of getting gestational diabetes by 26%.[2] Some good sources of fiber are Whole grains. Wheat bread, bulgur, oats, and quinoa all contain fiber. Fruit and veggie. Peas, corn, and broccoli are excellent suppliers, as are pears, blueberries, raspberries, and peaches. Consume the skins or peels for an additional dosage. Beans and legumes.

Fiber-rich legumes include lentils, black beans, kidney beans, lima beans, split peas, and chickpeas. Add them to stews or salads. Protein will assist your infant receive essential nutrients. Your protein requirements are determined by a variety of factors (including your level of activity) but aim for multiple servings distributed throughout the day. Plant-based options may include nuts, seeds, and legumes.

Protein-rich options include Fish. abundant-fat fish, such as salmon, are not only abundant in protein but also contain omega-3 fatty acids. Meat that is low in fat. Poultry (such as chicken or turkey) and lean beef are both suitable options. Black beans. One cup has 15 grams of protein. Use them to make breakfast burritos or homemade vegetable burgers.

What to eat when trying to get pregnant?
Here are some of the greatest meals to have on your plate when trying to conceive: Spinach. In general, aim for four to five servings of veggies per day.
Leafy greens, like spinach, are an excellent choice. Spinach is an excellent source of calcium, vitamin C, folate, and potassium. Add a handful of spinach leaves to your smoothie, along with vanilla yogurt and a ripe banana.

Oranges. Oranges also contain vitamin C, calcium, and potassium. Citrus fruits contain vitamin C, which can aid in the absorption of iron from non-meat sources. To incorporate more into your diet, try drinking orange juice or topping your salads with a few slices.

Milk. Dairy products provide protein, potassium, and calcium. Try to buy items that are enriched with vitamins A and D. Fortified milk can be used to make porridge or smoothies. Cereals are fortified. Whether you prefer prepared or ready-to-eat cereals, seek brands that are created from whole grains, fortified with iron and folic acid, and have less added sugar.

Chickpeas. Beans and peas are high in protein and also include iron and zinc. Chickpeas are particularly high in protein, zinc, potassium, and fiber. (Other acceptable possibilities are pinto beans, soybeans, white beans, lentils, and kidney beans.) They can be used to create hummus or baked and sprinkled over salads. Salmon. Salmon contains protein, omega-3 fatty acids, and potassium.

Healthy dietary suggestions for trying to get pregnant Overwhelmed? Do not be. You don't have to eat a "perfect" diet; simply tell yourself what you'll tell your child someday: do your best. And by prioritizing healthy eating habits now, you will find it simpler to maintain them once pregnant. When in doubt, consider these strategies:

Eat more fruits and vegetables. Produce contains high levels of vitamins A, C, iron, magnesium, potassium, and fiber. Aim for four to five servings of vegetables (at least two should be leafy greens) and three to four portions of fresh fruit every day. Check-in with an expert.

If you have any dietary limitations, such as being vegan or vegetarian or following a particular diet for a chronic condition, see your doctor about covering nutritional gaps in your meals. (A registered nutritionist can also assist.) If you feel you have an eating disorder, such as bulimia or anorexia nervosa, speak with your doctor about seeking the assistance of a health professional and a support group. Practice proper (food) hygiene. Food poisoning is hazardous to anyone, but it is more deadly if you are pregnant. Some foodborne infections can harm your baby's health even before conception.

Choose smart seafood. The Environmental Protection Agency (EPA) and the Food and Drug Administration (FDA) recommend that women who are attempting to conceive consume 8 to 12 ounces of low-mercury fish per week. Avoid seafood such as swordfish, tilefish, king mackerel, and shark. However, salmon, canned light tuna, cod, and shrimp are acceptable options.

Do not skip meals. You may choose to sleep through breakfast or work through lunch right now, but after a baby arrives, you'll require a consistent supply of nutrients throughout the day. Take a look at your calendar and make time for three full meals per day. Cut back on caffeine.

Despite popular belief, pregnant women can consume coffee; however, the American College of Obstetricians and Gynecologists (ACOG) and other organizations recommend that mothers-to-be limit their caffeine intake to no more than 200 mg per day or approximately one 12-ounce cup of coffee. If you usually order a grande or venti, consider limiting your caffeine intake now rather than later. Do not smoke. If you smoke, this is an excellent moment to quit. Tobacco use can make it difficult to conceive, and once pregnant, it can raise the risk of miscarriage.

Limit your alcohol intake. A few glasses of wine may make baby-making more joyful, but drinking too much can make it difficult to conceive. It's best to limit your alcohol consumption to a couple of glasses per week while you're trying, and completely abstain if you suspect you're pregnant because alcohol can harm a developing kid. Best to stick to a mocktail.

CHAPTER 4

FOODS TO AVOID WHEN TRYING TO CONCEIVE

Foods to avoid when trying to conceive. Are you trying to conceive but don't know which foods to avoid? There is no need to worry. We're here to tell you which meals to avoid when trying to conceive.

1. Quick meals. When trying to conceive, it is advised to avoid fast food because it can affect your fertility. Fast food has a lot of trans fat and processed sugar, both of which can cause hormonal problems. Eat nutrient-dense foods to boost your fertility. Fast eating causes weight gain, which may be the reason for your infertility. Avoid deep-fried foods to improve your overall health. Prioritize a well-balanced diet because it boosts fertility.

2. Foods High in Mercury You should avoid high-mercury foods like swordfish, king mackerel, and other fish since they can damage your fetus' growth. You may wonder why high-mercury foods should be avoided

while attempting to conceive. Mercury is a heavy element that is hazardous not only to embryonic growth but also to the neurological system and brain.

3. Foods high in sugar. Limit your intake of extremely sugary meals, which elevate your blood sugar levels. It also affects your reproductive health, raising your chances of getting polycystic ovary syndrome. These foods can induce hormonal imbalances and irregular menstrual cycles. Furthermore, consuming too much sugar can lower the quality of your eggs. Consuming sugary beverages lowers the likelihood of pregnancy.

4. Foods with high trans fat content. Foods high in trans fats and saturated fats can affect fertility. Trans fats can be found in animal products such as meat and dairy, as well as fast foods. Trans fats impair hormonal homeostasis and may cause ovulatory infertility. Consuming whole grains and cooking with healthy oils can help you become more fertile. When it comes to dairy foods, there may be a few ingredients that increase the risk of infection in your body while you are trying to conceive. Pasteurized dairy products can be replaced by nonpasteurized dairy products.

5. Foods that are undercooked Consuming undercooked and uncooked foods can increase your chances of being infected while trying to conceive. Heat raw meals

properly to reduce the risk of illness. Aside from undercooked and raw meals, you should avoid consuming too much soy because it disrupts hormone balance, so limit your intake. Excessive alcohol and caffeine use may result in reproductive difficulties. Caffeine use raises the risk of miscarriage; however, herbal tea can be drunk instead.

In contrast, alcohol increases the chance of infertility and reduces egg quality. It also leads to hormonal imbalances and disrupts the menstrual cycle. Certain meals should be avoided while attempting to conceive. To avoid pregnancy complications, you must first determine which foods to avoid. Avoiding fast food and eating a well-balanced diet will help you become fertile. Fast food contains a lot of dangerous chemicals and additives that are bad for your reproductive health.

CHAPTER 5

UNDERSTANDING MENSTRUAL CYCLE, FERTILITY, AND CONCEPTION

The first step toward becoming pregnant is to have sex and to do so regularly. However, to increase your monthly chances of conception, you must first discover the optimal times to get intimate. Women's menstrual cycles have various phases.

Each woman's cycle is unique, but understanding what's going on in your body might help you boost your chances of having a kid. Your Menstrual Cycle The menstrual cycle begins with the formation of 10 to 20 eggs, which stimulates the production of the female hormone estrogen. It makes the uterine lining thicken in preparation for a prospective pregnancy.

Ovulation happens when one or more eggs mature and the ovary discharges them into the fallopian tubes. If there is no sperm to fertilize the egg, it will die within 12 to 24 hours. However, if sperm is present when the egg is released, it may fertilize the egg, and if the embryo attaches to the uterus, a pregnancy can begin. Following ovulation, your body produces a second hormone, progesterone, which strengthens the uterine lining and helps support a pregnancy.

If no pregnancy occurs, the uterine lining breaks down, resulting in a monthly cycle. Your most fruitful days. So, keeping your menstrual cycle in mind, you may begin to grasp why timing is critical for getting pregnant. Your most fertile days are the three days preceding and including ovulation.

It is possible to become pregnant if you have sex within five days after ovulation or on the day of ovulation, as sperm can live for up to five days. The window closes between 12 and 24 hours following ovulation. So, how do you know you're ovulating? You might start by evaluating your monthly cycle. The first day of your period is called "day one" of your cycle.

Ovulation occurs approximately 14 days before the start of your period, so you may make an accurate approximation if you know the usual length of your monthly cycle. For example, if your monthly cycle lasts 28 days on average, your most fertile days will be

12-13-14. Ovulation trackers, available both online and as apps, can help you track your cycles and estimate your most fertile days.

When you're ovulating, you should also be aware of several bodily indicators. During your most fertile period, your cervical mucus often grows thinner, clearer, wetter, and more slippery. You can also buy an ovulation predictor kit at a supermarket or pharmacist, which uses urine tests to determine when you will ovulate.

The chances of falling pregnant According to statistics, the average woman who has intercourse five days before ovulation has a 10% chance of becoming pregnant, which increases to 30% if a woman has sex on the day of ovulation or two days prior. These figures will vary according to a woman's age. If you're not sure when you're ovulating, most doctors recommend having sex every two to three days to increase your chances of becoming pregnant.

Despite feeling healthy and enjoying regular intercourse, you may not become pregnant. Women and their spouses may experience mental distress and difficulty when dealing with pregnancy delay or infertility. Doctors urge that if you are under 35 and have been trying to conceive unsuccessfully for 12 months or longer, you consult a GP or specialist. If you are over 35, it is recommended that you seek help after six months of attempting to conceive.

CHAPTER 6

HEALTHY SPERM: IMPROVING FERTILITY

Healthy sperm is not always a given. Understand how lifestyle influences your sperm and what you can do to increase your fertility. People considering a pregnancy may be concerned about the health of their sperm. Understand what factors can influence male fertility, and then examine how to help the sperm attain the goal.

Male Reproductive System What causes sperm health? Sperm health depends on several characteristics, including quantity, motility, and structure: Quantity. Fertility is most likely when the semen released in a single ejaculation (ejaculate) contains at least 15 million sperm per milliliter. Too little sperm in ejaculation may make it more difficult to become pregnant since there are fewer candidates available to fertilize the egg. Movement.

To reach and fertilize an egg, sperm must travel through the female cervix, uterus, and fallopian tubes. This is referred to as motility. Pregnancy can occur with fewer than 40% of the sperm in the ejaculate moving, but 40% is regarded as the threshold. More is better. Morphology, or structure.

Typical sperm have oval heads and long tails that combine to propel them. This is less crucial than the quantity or mobility of sperm. What causes male fertility issues? Several medical disorders can lead to male fertility problems, including A disorder in the hypothalamus or pituitary gland, regions of the brain that stimulate the testicles to generate testosterone and sperm (secondary hypogonadism). Testicular disease.

Disorders of sperm transport. Age can also play a part. Sperm motility and the number of normal sperm decline with age, decreasing fertility, particularly after the age of 50.

What is the greatest approach to creating healthy sperm? To boost the chances of creating healthy sperm, take the following simple steps: Maintain a healthy body weight. According to some research, increasing body mass index (BMI) is associated with a decrease in sperm count and motility. Eat a nutritious diet.

Choose a variety of fruits and vegetables, which are high in antioxidants and may help increase sperm quality. Prevent STIs. Sexually transmitted illnesses, such as chlamydia and gonorrhea, can cause infertility in men.

Limiting the number of sexual partners and always using a condom for sex — or remaining in a mutually monogamous relationship with an uninfected partner — can aid in STI prevention. Manage your stress. Stress can impair sexual function and disrupt the hormones required to make sperm. Start moving. Moderate physical activity can boost the amounts of potent antioxidant enzymes that help protect sperm.

What's off-limits? Sperm can be particularly vulnerable to environmental conditions such as high temperatures or harmful chemicals. To preserve fertility:

Do not smoke. Men who smoke cigarettes have lower sperm counts. If you smoke, seek your doctor for help quitting.

Limit your alcohol intake. Heavy drinking can cause low testosterone levels, impotence, and decreased sperm production. If you choose to drink, do so moderately. For healthy people, this equates to one drink per day for women and two drinks per day for men.

Avoid using lubricants during sex. While more research is needed to determine the effects of lubricants on fertility, consider avoiding them during intercourse. If necessary, use mineral oil, canola oil, mustard oil, or a fertility-friendly lubricant like Pre-Seed. Consult a health care practitioner about drugs. Calcium channel blockers, tricyclic antidepressants, anti-androgens, opioids, and other drugs can all lead to fertility difficulties.

Anabolic steroids and other illegal medications can provide the same effects.

Take precautions against poisons. Pesticides, lead, and other pollutants can impair sperm quantity and quality. If you have to work with poisons, do so safely.

Wear protective clothing, utilize protective equipment, such as safety goggles, and keep chemicals away from your skin. Keep it cool. Increased scrotal temperature can reduce sperm production. Although the benefits have not been fully demonstrated, wearing loose-fitting underwear, sitting less, avoiding saunas and hot pools, and limiting scrotum exposure to heated things, such as a laptop, may improve sperm quality. Chemotherapy and radiation therapy for cancer can decrease sperm production and produce infertility that may be permanent.

Consult a healthcare practitioner about the possibilities of extracting and conserving sperm before treatment. When is it time to seek help? Adopting healthy lifestyle choices to support fertility — and avoiding items that can harm it — can increase the likelihood of conceiving. If you and your partner haven't gotten pregnant after a year of unprotected intercourse, you might consider getting tested for infertility. A fertility specialist may be able to determine the source of the problem and provide therapies that will put you and your partner on the path to motherhood.

CHAPTER 7

HOW TO IMPROVE EGG QUALITY

The phrase "egg quality" refers to whether an egg is genetically normal (euploid) or aberrant (aneuploid). All of a woman's eggs (approximately one or two million) are present at birth, and one of them matures each month, ready for ovulation.

The egg begins to mature when it is selected for ovulation. The process of producing a healthy child is prone to error as eggs age, resulting in the presence of abnormal DNA and prohibiting the egg from performing its original job.

High-quality eggs promote strong embryo growth and are essential for successful sperm fertilization. A high-quality egg increases the likelihood of the embryo implanting into the uterus. In other words, successful pregnancies result from higher-quality eggs producing higher-quality embryos.

A high-quality, healthy egg must have the appropriate amount of chromosomes and be able to fuse with sperm. Signs of Good and Poor Quality Eggs In the context of fertility, female egg quality refers to the health and developmental potential of a woman's eggs or ova. It is a critical factor that influences the chances of a healthy pregnancy and successful conception. Signs of Good Quality Eggs High-quality eggs boost the chances that they will be fertilized, develop into an embryo, or implant, and result in pregnancy. Fertility is dependent on healthy eggs, which contain the genetic material essential for embryo development.

A chromosomally faulty egg will not always fertilize, and if it does, it may generate an abnormal embryo that will either implant normally or, in the worst-case scenario, cause a miscarriage or produce a sick child. Thus, "good egg quality" is associated with higher rates of fertilization, higher-quality embryos, and a better chance of successful implantation.

Signs of high-quality eggs include: Balanced hormone levels Regular menstrual periods Variations in the body's basal temperature and cervical fluid levels occur throughout the menstrual cycle. A healthy egg or ovum with normal genetic makeup contains 23 chromosomes (euploid). An egg with a chromosomal aberration (aneuploid) contains fewer or more chromosomes than

23. This leads to poor egg quality and the development of genetic defects following fertilization. Signs of Poor-Quality Egg Poor-quality eggs can make conception difficult, increase the risk of miscarriage, and diminish the chances of a successful pregnancy. Signs of low-quality eggs include Hormonal abnormalities that may produce irregular or inconsistent menstrual periods, affecting egg quality. An abnormal chromosome count could be a sign of poor egg quality.

Aberrant or low-quality eggs will have fewer or more chromosomes than normal. Because chromosomally damaged embryos are more likely to miscarry, several miscarriages could suggest low-quality eggs. Low levels of follicle-stimulating hormone (FSH) may indicate diminishing egg quality. FSH is a hormone produced by the pituitary gland that directs the ovaries to release one egg each cycle. Infertility treatments that consistently result in low egg production or low fertility rates may suggest a problem with the quality of the eggs generated.

Low estrogen levels are another sign of low egg quality. Estradiol is the hormone that transmits messages from the ovaries to the brain. Reduced anti-mullerian hormone (AMH) levels could indicate poor egg quality. AMH is a glycoprotein produced by egg cells during their early developing stage. It promotes the development and maturity of eggs. If you are having problems with egg quality, contact the top IVF hospital in Kerala. They will help you improve egg quality for your parenting journey.

What Causes Poor-Quality Eggs?
The quality of the egg naturally deteriorates with age. However, other factors contribute to women's infertility and poor egg quality. Understanding the root causes is critical for resolving the problem.

Here are a few proven reasons why eggs aren't of excellent quality:
Age The quality of eggs is substantially impacted by their age. Age-related decreases in egg production may raise the possibility that the surviving eggs contain genetic defects. Fertility decreases after the age of 35. Autoimmune disorders. An inflammatory attack on the ovaries might have a negative influence on egg quality as well as ovarian reserve.

Genetic disorders An inherited tendency might also contribute to poor egg quality. Certain genetic conditions can alter the quality of eggs produced. Lifestyle and Environment Smoking, heavy drinking, being overweight, and exposure to environmental toxins can all have an impact on egg quality.

Tubercular Disorders Tubal diseases are regarded as one of the most common causes of reduced egg quality and infertility in women. Radiation and Chemotherapy Radiation therapy at high doses has the potential to decrease egg quality and perhaps cause early menopause. According to a study, chemotherapy can cause the ovaries to stop releasing estrogen and eggs. Endometriosis This condition decreases egg quality when tissue resembling the uterine lining grows outside of it, near other reproductive organs such as the ovaries.

How Can I Improve Egg Quality?
Here are some strategies to improve the quality of your eggs for IVF or pregnancy. Eat a healthy diet. One strategy for producing high-quality eggs is to be in generally good health. It is influenced by your eating and drinking habits. According to studies, eating a diet rich in fruits, vegetables, and other nutrients can improve fertility.

Make sure all of the foods in your diet are nutritional; avoid processed, sugary, and high-saturated fat foods. In addition to eating a healthy diet, taking vitamins that aid in egg production is recommended. Fish oil, vitamins A and E, and melatonin all help to increase egg quality. Achieve a normal BMI. A normal BMI can enhance the chances of becoming pregnant. Obesity has been linked to reduced egg quality and increased oxidative stress on your cells. Increase Blood Flow.

Healthy egg production is dependent on the ovaries obtaining oxygen-rich blood. It is critical to maintain sufficient hydration to increase oxygenated blood flow to these tissues. Drink six to eight glasses of water or other fluids every day, at minimum. Exercise is essential for improving circulation throughout the body and increasing blood flow to the heart. Furthermore, massage therapy and yoga promote blood flow.

Stress can disturb ovulation by releasing hormones such as prolactin and cortisol, leading to reduced egg production. Stress can promote the release of hormones such as prolactin and cortisol, disrupting or stopping ovulation and reducing egg production. Stay away from smoking and drinking. Women who are attempting to conceive or are undergoing IVF should avoid smoking. Women who are attempting to conceive or are undergoing IVF should avoid smoking.

Furthermore, these cigarettes include harmful substances that change the DNA of egg cells, making them inefficient for pregnancy. Because women generate fewer eggs as they age, it is better to preserve viable eggs safe from potentially harmful toxins. Reduce your consumption of alcohol and caffeine, as these may have an impact on your fertility.

What Diet Can Help to Improve Egg Quality?

The foods you eat have a significant impact on your entire health, including your energy, emotions, and fertility. Your body uses nutrients from your meals and supplements to build hormones, repair cells, and finally produce healthy eggs. Your food choices have a big effect on your fertility.

The following foods are typically recommended to promote reproductive health and egg quality: Add leafy greens to your diet, such as Swiss chard, kale, spinach, and fenugreek. Include some colorful fruits and vegetables, such as broccoli, oranges, bell peppers, and berries. Walnuts, chia seeds, flaxseeds, and fatty fish (sardines, salmon) are all good sources of omega-3 fatty acids. These meals can also help to balance hormones and minimize inflammation. Include protein-rich meals including fish, chicken, eggs, lentils, tofu, and lean meats.

Choose whole grains rich in fiber and essential nutrients, such as quinoa, brown rice, oats, and whole wheat bread. Include heart-healthy fats such as nuts, seeds, avocados, and olive oil. These fats aid in the production of hormones and provide essential nutrients. Antioxidants present in berries, citrus fruits, tomatoes, and green tea protect eggs from oxidative stress and improve reproductive health in general.

When looking for ways to improve the quality of your eggs, add fermented foods like yogurt to your diet. They increase nutrient absorption and support gut health. Is it possible to improve egg quality in 30 days? An egg takes approximately three months or ninety days to mature from an immature oocyte to an egg ready for ovulation. Thus, three months before conception is the optimal period to undertake dietary and lifestyle changes that will improve egg quality. That being said, this doesn't mean you won't get results sooner. Moving forward, the changes you make here will benefit all aspects of your fertility, not simply the quality of your eggs. Everything contributes to increasing your chances of becoming pregnant and having a healthy pregnancy. It is critical for women trying to conceive to understand how to improve the quality of their eggs.

It is feasible to enhance egg quality in 30 days by eating fertility-friendly foods, taking supplements, and modifying your lifestyle. By being proactive, you can improve the quality of your eggs. Conclusion Understanding the significance of egg quality is an important step on your path to parenting. It may require some time and effort to increase the quality of your eggs. However, you can increase your chances of becoming pregnant by using fertility drugs, and supplements, and making appropriate lifestyle changes.

CHAPTER 8

LIFESTYLE FACTORS AND THEIR EFFECT ON FERTILITY

Infertility is a widespread condition that affects people of all income levels and races. Infertility affects 9-30% of the population in low-income countries and 15% in high-income countries, thus it cannot be disregarded. Infertility is medically defined as the failure to conceive after twelve months of unprotected intercourse. It can be caused by a variety of causes.

The effects of numerous lifestyle factors on fertility, such as smoking, nutrition, exercise, substance use, chemical exposures, stress, and delayed childbirth. Medical disorders that contribute to male and female infertility are also mentioned. Smoking Smoking has a deleterious influence on both male and female fertility.

In men, oxidative stress can affect sperm production, motility, and morphology while also increasing the chance of DNA damage. Smoking can also affect luteal hormone levels, fallopian tube contraction, sperm-egg contact, and oocyte transfer. Cigarette smoke metabolites can be identified in women whose spouses smoke.

These metabolites influence ovarian follicle growth as well as the fallopian tubes, which contributes to ectopic pregnancy. Weight, Diet, and Exercise. Being underweight or overweight might hurt fertility. Obese women have decreased amounts of sex hormone-binding globulin (SHBG), which typically binds hormones such as testosterone. Obesity also increases women's risk of gestational diabetes and hypertension. Men with a body mass index (BMI) outside of the normal weight range may have low sperm quality. Adipose tissue secretions hamper spermatogenesis and produce more reactive oxygen species.

A good diet, weight loss, and exercise can all boost fertility in both men and women. However, exercise should be done in moderation; overdoing it can strain the body and affect fertility. Coffee and Alcohol Caffeine and alcohol consumption have been linked to longer conception times. Although contentious, research has shown that excessive coffee drinking affects hormone levels in the body, increases the risk of miscarriage, and is connected with low birth weight.

The link between drinking and birth abnormalities is well documented. While the exact amount of alcohol required to have these negative effects is debatable, chronic alcohol intake impairs fertility in both men and women.

Environmental Pollutants and Oncofertility Environmental contaminants including radiation, pesticides, and phthalates can all cause infertility.

Cancer and its accompanying treatments can have a significant impact on fertility. People diagnosed with cancer at a young age should address their fertility early on and monitor it constantly over time.

Psychological Stress Stress, like amenorrhea, can have a substantial impact on fertility. A stressful job may reduce a woman's chances of conceiving, and a heavy workload reduces the chances of successfully finishing a pregnancy.

Stress has been linked to a decrease in sperm count and motility in men. Delayed childbearing In an increasingly profession-driven environment, many women prefer to pursue a career before starting a family. This has resulted in a delay in the age when women consider having children. Fertility reduces with age beginning around age 32, so by the time a woman has established her profession, she may find it more difficult to conceive. This discovery can be upsetting because she now has a limited time before she becomes infertile due to age.

Delaying conception may raise the chance of spontaneous abortion, miscarriage, and congenital abnormalities. This age-related drop in fertility is not exclusive to women. Men have a drop in fertility as they age, though not as dramatically as women. Men are more likely to suffer from damage, cancer, and inflammation in their reproductive organs as they age. They may also experience lower testosterone levels.

Additionally, up to 40% of males with infertility may have a varicocele, which is an abnormal distention of the testicular venous plexus. These causes could all lead to male infertility. Medical Conditions Affecting Fertility Infertility can be caused by a variety of medical disorders. Secondary hypothalamic amenorrhea occurs when the hypothalamus and pituitary gland communicate ineffectively, limiting fertility.

Chronic stress can be the source of the illness if the body is unable to adapt properly to stress. Without adaptation, gonadotropins are decreased and unable to successfully stimulate the menstrual cycle. Another medical disorder that affects fertility is polycystic ovarian syndrome (PCOS). Infertility affects one out of every four women with PCOS, and other symptoms include irregular periods, anovulation, hyperandrogenism, weight gain, and insulin resistance.

Asymptomatic uterine myomas (fibroids) can potentially reduce fertility. These benign uterine tumors may cause issues in the future as they accumulate and expand. This may result in irregular bleeding and reduced uterine contractility. Myomas have been linked to an increased risk of miscarriage, premature birth, and other pregnancy problems. Endometriosis is another cause of infertility, as it can cause dysmenorrhea, pelvic pain, and stomach pain.

Endometriosis is strongly associated with infertility. According to some research, 30-50% of women with infertility have endometriosis, and infertile women are 6-8 times more likely to have it. Several hypothesized mechanisms investigate the effects of endometriosis on fertility. One reason could be an inflammatory milieu that hinders sperm-egg contact, while others suggest adhesions that disrupt oocyte descent, ovarian reserve depletion, and impaired endometrial receptivity.

www.ingramcontent.com/pod-product-compliance
Lightning Source LLC
Chambersburg PA
CBHW051713250726
48653CB00007B/3016